Resistance Workout for Seniors

Complete Guide to Resistance Band Workouts for Seniors

Introduction

Are you a senior looking to learn more about resistance band workouts, a type of exercise that, besides being one of the most senior-friendly, can also change how you view exercise and is fun to integrate into your daily routine?

If yes, keep reading:

This guidebook is going to give you all the information you need to know about resistance band workouts, including:

- What resistance band workouts are

- The benefits of resistance band workouts

- How to choose a resistance band that is ideal for you

- How to warm up before a resistance band workout

- The different types of resistant band workouts for seniors,

- And different resistance band-based workouts for various conditions such as back pain, diabetes, osteoporosis, hip, knee, and shoulder issues

- And so much more:

There's no doubt that if you're a senior looking to get started with resistance band exercises, you will find this book valuable and actionable!

Let's begin!

Table of Content

Introduction _____ 2

Section 1 _____ 8

Introduction to Resistance Band Workout 8

    Resistance Band Defined _____ 8

    Benefits of Using Resistance Bands _____ 9

    How To Choose a Suitable Band _____ 12

    Safe Usage: Resistance Band Usage Tips _____ 17

Section 2 _____ 21

Warm-Ups and Stretches _____ 21

    Warm-Up Activities _____ 22

    Common Warming-Up Mistakes_____ 23

    The Warm-Up Routines _____ 25

    Stretching Routines _____ 40

Section 3 _____ 65

Resistance Band Workout Guidelines ___ **65**

Section 4 _____ **70**

Resistance Band Workout Exercises For Seniors _____ **70**

    Upper Body Exercises_____ 70

Lower Body Exercises _____ **84**

Abdominal Exercises _____ **94**

Chest Exercises _____ **100**

Shoulder Exercises _____ **102**

Back Exercises _____ **108**

Thigh Exercises _____ **110**

Glute and Hip Flexor Exercises _____ **114**

Calf Exercise _____ **122**

Section 5 _____ **123**

Cooling Down _____ 123

Section 6 _____ 131

Resistance Band Workout Programs ____ 131

    What to Keep In Mind When Designing a Personal Resistance Band Training Program _____ 133

Beginner's Workout Program _____ 135

Arthritis Workout Program _____ 139

Back Pain Workout Program _____ 143

Hip Issues Workout Program _____ 147

Knee Issues Workout Program _____ 150

Osteoporosis Workout Program _____ 153

Shoulder Issues Workout Program _____ 156

Diabetes Workout Program _____ 159

High Blood Pressure Program _____ 162

Conclusion _____ **166**

Section 1

Introduction to Resistance Band Workout

To understand resistance band workouts, you need to understand what a resistance band is.

Resistance Band Defined

A resistance band is an elastic, rope-like piece of rubber band specially designed for resistance-driven exercises. There are many different types of resistance bands, and in a later section, we shall discuss what to look for when purchasing a resistance band.

Resistance band workouts exploit the resistance applied by resistance bands when you try to stretch them, subsequently exerting a level of strain on your muscles. The energy you muster to oppose this resistance creates endurance in your muscles over time, which is the primary concept behind the effectiveness of resistance band workouts.

Resistance bands are some of the most effective workout tools in existence, and the benefits of workouts that integrate the use of these tools are many:

Benefits of Using Resistance Bands

Now that you know what resistance bands are, you are probably asking yourself:

"Why should I integrate these bands into my workout routine?"

Well, the reasons are several:

First, these bands are easy to carry around. Moreover, they don't require much space to use or store, which is not something we can say for other exercise tools such as dumbbells and other gym tools.

Secondly, resistance bands have varying resistance levels and are easy to exchange once you get stronger and feel the need for a band of stronger resistance.

Third, resistance band workouts only require 10 to 15 minutes a day, and they are suitable for everyone, which makes them adaptable. Whether you are a senior, a convalescent, or a top-tier athlete, the resistance band has a workout routine or exercise in store for you. This form of working out might even offer more benefits than conventional strength training using gym weights.

Some of the other benefits of integrating resistance band workouts into your daily routine include:

#: *Slows cell deterioration*

Cells Deterioration is more or less the rate at which your cells age (rate of aging).

If the rate at which your old cells are dying is higher than the rate at which your body produces new cells to replace them, it means you are growing old relatively faster. While old age is inevitable, you can slow down the process a little so that you won't lose a lot of your muscle energy as you age.

Resistance band workouts help slow the aging process, which ensures that you can remain healthier for longer.

A 2011 study that appeared in the journal *Sports Medicine* investigated the [effects of resistance training in the muscles of older adults](). The study concluded that such workouts slowed down the aging process. Further research even showed that besides slowing down the aging process, such exercises could also reverse the effects of aging.

#: It can help manage arthritis

If you have arthritis, then resistance band workouts are going to prove immensely beneficial, which is why physical therapists often recommend this form of exercise as a way to combat the condition. For instance, on [their blog,](#) the Arthritis Foundation lists resistance bands as one of the ways to ease symptoms of the condition.

On its part, from an investigative survey, the [Journal of Rheumatology concluded that four months of resistance training](#), those suffering from knee arthritis experienced a 42% in pain reduction and a 44% increase in physical function and mobility.

#: It reduces the chances of injury

Resistance band workouts can strengthen your bones and make them denser. According to [Mayo Clinic](#), it does this by stressing the bones, making them compact and slightly bigger. Enhanced bone strength and density make you less susceptible to injury, even after a fall.

Resistance band workout can also help improve your stability, hence reducing your chances of falling. Unlike other forms of exercise, using the bands themselves has a minimal risk of injury.

It can boost your mood

Whenever you engage in a workout routine, the body releases chemicals called endorphins. These chemicals interact with neuron receptors in your brain, a process that generates a feeling of happiness by stifling your perception of pain.

Resistance band workouts can convert you into a walking dispenser of feel-good hormones. The change will be noticeable—to you and others— and can significantly improve your quality of life.

Having looked at the benefits of resistance band workouts, let's discuss what you need to keep in mind when choosing a resistance band:

How To Choose a Suitable Band

Resistance bands have differing intensities. Your muscle tone and skill level will determine which type of band you get. However, worth noting is that you do not necessarily have to buy a single band. Many sellers and manufacturers sell resistance bands as a set made up of bands of different resistance levels.

Keep in mind that different workout routines might require varying bands depending on the resistance force. For instance, when exercising your legs, you might need a band that's different from the one you'd use when working out your hands. Because of the varying resistances, purchasing a full set starter kit is the best way to go.

Many sellers and manufacturers sell resistance bands, many of which you can find online. In most cases, they color-code their bands according to their resistance strength. The color codes are universal, and one of the popular makers of resistance bands, Theraband, has the bands available in the colors shown in the image below.

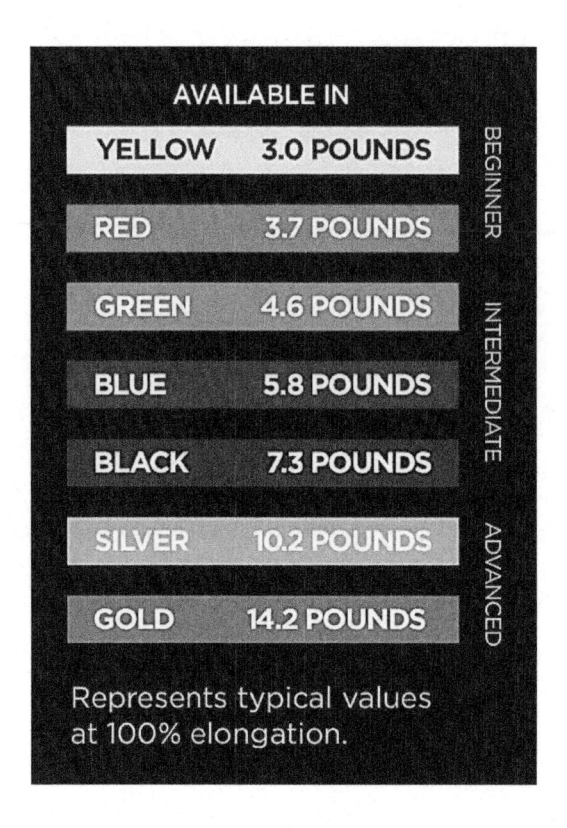

AVAILABLE IN		
YELLOW	3.0 POUNDS	BEGINNER
RED	3.7 POUNDS	
GREEN	4.6 POUNDS	INTERMEDIATE
BLUE	5.8 POUNDS	
BLACK	7.3 POUNDS	
SILVER	10.2 POUNDS	ADVANCED
GOLD	14.2 POUNDS	

Represents typical values at 100% elongation.

Image 1: The Color Codes, courtesy of TheraBand

What the Colours Mean

When you pick up resistance bands, what you will quickly notice when you try to get a feel for them by stretching is their different resistance levels. Generally, the bands fall into three categories: Light, Medium, and Heavy resistance bands, based on their resistance strength.

As a senior, most of the time, you are going to use the beginner and intermediate level resistance bands. These are the bands used to exercise smaller muscles group like the hips and shoulder. Thus, the yellow and red bands are the ideal choice for you as a beginner and senior.

At the medium level, we have green, blue and black bands. As you continue exercising, you'll become stronger, and should consider integrating bands at this level to your fitness routine. The mid-tier bands are also the bands you want to use to exercise stronger muscles of your body like the back, legs, and chest.

To make it easier to understand what the resistance level represents, think of them as forces or weights. The image above shows the force a resistance band exerts when stretched to twice its length. This force is in weight form, which can help you roughly gauge how that would feel.

Color	Resistance	Muscle Group
Yellow	Extra Light	Shoulders and Shins
Red	Light	Biceps and Triceps
Green	Medium	Legs, Chest & Back

| Blue | Medium/Heavy | Legs, Chest & Back |

Table 1: Bands and the muscles groups they work out best for seniors

As you continue using your new set of bands as part of your fitness routine, you will start to get a feel for which bands work best for which workout and muscle group.

When it comes to resistance training, getting the resistance right is a trial and error matter, and thus, what is best for you might not be best for the next person.

If you listen to your body as you work out, you will eventually learn your new bands and shall be able to know each band based on its unique, innate qualities and resistance.

If we consider their shape, there're two main types of resistance bands: flat and tubular.

If this is your first time engaging in resistance bands, it's best to begin with the flat type and then work your way up from there. If you are allergic to latex, keep in mind that some manufacturers make latex-free, flat variant resistance bands that you can use.

Today, tubular type of resistance bands are gradually gaining popularity because of their durability and the fact that they come with extra features like padded handles. Some of them have adjustable handles that allow you to lengthen or shorten the band to fit your size.

The other thing you need to know is how to use these resistance bands to derive the best effect from them:

Safe Usage: Resistance Band Usage Tips

This guide aims to supply you with relevant resistance band workouts information, not as a substitute for a professional instructor or trainer. Before you integrate resistance band workouts into your work out routine, consult your general physician or trainer:

With that out of the way, it is worth noting that there are a few things you should be watchful of when you decide to use resistance bands to exercise. That's because although resistance bands are widely safe to use as a workout tool, it is always advisable to consult your doctor before you start any form of workout.

That notwithstanding, if you adhere to the following general safety tips, you should be okay;

- **Always pay attention to your body**: For example, one morning, you might wake up with a pain in your left elbow, in which case, engaging in arm-based workouts would be detrimental to your wellbeing. Remember not to subject your body to any load until you feel better again.

- **Warm-up:** Always engage in warm-up exercises before you start using your resistance bands or engage in any work out for that matter. Additionally, stretch your body at the end of every workout session. Many of those new to working out, often out of eagerness and over-zealousness, dive into the deep end, which can prove costly. Remember that it's better to be safe than sorry. Take your time and ease yourself into a manageable, consistent workout routine.

- **Watch out for allergies:** If you are allergic to latex, do not use latex-based resistance bands. Instead, purchase latex-free resistance bands; you'll find many options at online stores.

- **Shoes:** Before you begin working out, wear nice-fitting, non-slip shoes; it will help you avoid slipping during work out routines.

- **Release tension:** Under no circumstance should you release the band while you have it stretched or under tension; doing so could be potentially risky. The band builds up energy as you stretch it. When you let go of one end while the resistance band is in this state, it could snap and strike you or anyone around you and cause serious injury.

- **Inspect:** Always inspect the band for any cracks, splits, or tears to make sure the band won't break in the middle of your workout session. If you find a defective or deformed band, do not use it.

- **Jewelry:** Take off any loose jewelry that might entangle with the band as you exercise, especially chains and necklaces.

- **Store your bands well:** Please do not store your bands in storage places that expose them to ultraviolet rays, high temperatures, oils, or solvents. These conditions affect the structural integrity of the bands and can cause rapid wear and tear. Note too that hand oils and lotions will damage your bands and cause rapid deterioration. These substances cause latex to crack and break. Therefore, before using your resistance bands, error on the safe side, and wash your hands well.

- **Breath:** Get into the habit of breathing through exercises. Breathe deeply and avoid holding your breath, especially through the difficult parts. If you hold your breath during a work out routine, it will cause you to feel drowsy, which might lead to tension headaches and muscle burnout. Deep breathing helps send more oxygen to your blood for circulation, which is what you want because, during workouts, your muscles need plenty of oxygen to avoid burning out.

If you keep these general usage tips in mind, you should be able to use resistance bands safely.

As mentioned, this book only seeks to complement your physician's advice. Before you embark on any workout regimen, including the resistance band workout routines in this guide, consult your physician.

One of the most important things you should do before you workout using resistance bands is to warm up. Let's discuss that in the next section:

Section 2

Warm-Ups and Stretches

As stated earlier, warming up is a critical part of any workout routine, and is something we cannot overemphasize, especially for seniors. Exercising when your muscles are cold increases the risk of injuries and muscle tears.

Your body is like a machine that, to keep functioning optimally, requires maintenance and good care. If a car's engine needs a little warming up before it can start performing at its optimum level, it should tell you that your body needs warming up too before it can perform exercise routines at its optimum level.

The objective behind warming is to promote respiration and to increase your core body temperature and blood circulation to your muscles to ready them for the impending workout.

If you don't know which activities or exercises to engage in as part of your warm-up routine, this section will help you with that.

Warm-Up Activities

Warming-up is so simple that it does not require any machinery. Don't overcomplicate it, because regular, day-to-day activities can be part of your warm-up routine.

You can even perform the following activities before your workout session as part of your workout routine.

- Go for a walk (at a faster-than-normal pace)
- Ride your bike a few times around the block
- Dance around, twist and shake your body (any vigorous movement that warms your body will do fine)
- Walk up and down the stairs

Before we start discussing specific warm-up routines you can engage in before your main resistance band fitness routine, let's discuss some common warm-up mistakes you should avoid:

Common Warming-Up Mistakes

Avoid the following warm-up mistakes:

#: *Not warming up*

Failing to warm-up is the number one mistake you should avoid.

When you first resolve to work out, out of eagerness, you may want to get into the working out part immediately, assuming it's the part that is going to give you the results you want. Don't be one of those people.

Be patient and treat this as a process, which is what it is.

#: *Not stretching*

Some people warm up but forget to stretch. Many people ignore stretching because of the wrong perception that there is no gain without pain.

There is no pain in stretching, yes, but that's the beauty of it: you gain something, minus the pain. Do not skip this vital stage before you start your resistance band workout routine.

#: Holding static stretches for too long

Hold stretches for only as long as you don't feel any strain or pain. As soon as you begin to feel any discomfort, stop!

#: Under-stimulation or over-fatigue

Doing less than required to warm is just as bad as overdoing it. A balance is crucial; it ensures your body does not breakdown.

The Warm-Up Routines

This section is going to describe warm-up exercises you can do anywhere. These warm-up exercises are an excellent way to get your muscles ready for the next phase of your workout, which is the stretching phase.

They can also help prevent injury, which is why you should get into a habit of doing them every time you are about to take on a work out routine. You can even perform these exercises as a way to start your day and body juices flowing.

#: Marching and swinging arms

To carry out this exercise,

- Stand with your feet slightly apart. Relax your hands and keep them in position by the side of your body, not touching the trunk of your body. They shall be hanging free and forming the letter "V" upside down.

- Raise your right leg off the ground up to a level where your knee bend makes a 90-degree angle as you are marching. As you do this, inhale deeply through your nose.

- Drop your right leg, and as soon as it hits the ground, lift your left to make a 90-degree angle at your knee bend. Make sure you check your breathing and keep it in rhythm. As your left leg is lifting off the ground, you should exhale through your mouth.

- Keep up with this marching motion for about 5 seconds before you introduce another set of motion that puts your idle hands to action.

- While still marching with your hands in the upside-down V position, start swinging your hands. Bring your hands forward and crisscross them in front of your body and then bring them behind in a swinging motion.

- Remember to maintain a steady breathing pattern.

- Keep swinging and marching for the desired amount of time—2-10 minutes should do.

#: *Jog in Place*

This exercise involves jogging but not making any ground. Stick to your position and do light skipping up and down. As you jog in place, observe the following tips:

- Breath in through the nose and out through the mouth.

- Work out your hands and make them swing at the joint with your upper body.

- Keep your joint at the elbow moving.

- Keep this up for your desired amount of time—2-10 minutes.

#: *Jumping jacks*

This exercise works your lungs, heart, and muscles at the same time. The specific target muscles are glutes, quadriceps, and hip flexors. It also involves your abdominal and shoulder muscles.

Jumping jacks make your movements more explosive, adding to your strength and agility so you can achieve multidirectional movement with ease. According to [this study](), this warm-up exercise can also give you denser bones.

Results from a [research study]() suggest that everyone can perform this exercise safely, including children and older adults. However, if you have issues with your joints, injuries, or any health concerns, consult your doctor.

To perform jumping jacks, follow the steps below:

- Begin with standing up straight in the proper posture, with your legs together and arms resting on your hips.

- Bend your knees a little and jump slightly into the air. The higher, the more intense the exercise is going to be.

- Spread your legs apart to form an upside-down V as you toss yourself into the air.

- Stretch your arm wide apart and over your head in midair at the peak of your jump.

- Bring your legs back together as you fall back on to the ground and resume your original position.

- Repeat as many times as desired.

#: *Walking Jacks*

Walking jacks are ideal if you cannot do the jumping jacks—they are an alternative to jumping jacks. Here's how to do it:

- Start this exercise by standing in proper posture, sticking your chest out, and maintaining good balance.

- Using your right leg, step out wide to the right. As you do this, simultaneously swing your arms out and over the top of your head. Swing your arms the same way you would when performing jumping jacks.

- Once you have the right foot firmly fixed on the ground, follow it by stepping the left leg in to bring your two legs together. Swing the arms back down and back to your original position. As you are doing all this, remember to breathe in and out.

- When you get the rhythm, you can start making the steps faster to get even more out of this exercise.

#: *March With Pull Down*

Here how to perform this warm-up exercise:

- Start by standing in the proper posture, your back straightened, abs tightened, your shoulders relaxed, and feet spread out shoulder-width.

- Raise your hands straight and parallel to each other on top of your head and pointing to the ceiling.

- As you pull your right foot off the ground to make that 90-degree angle at your knee joint, inhale through your mouth as deeply as you can. While doing this, simultaneously pull down both your hands and bring your elbow to the sides of your body.

- Return your right leg to the ground as you charge both your hands back into the air, pointing to the ceiling.

- Switch sides, and this time, lift your left foot off the ground, making a marching movement and pulling down your hands at the same time.

- Repeat this over the desired number of times.

To enhance the effectiveness of this exercise, observe the following tips:

- Before engaging in this exercise, master the marching in place movement.

- Do not lean back each you lift your knees.

- To make the exercise more intense, march faster, and raise your knees higher.

#: *Lateral Step*

To perform the lateral step:

- Stand straight, then, take your right leg and move it behind your right leg, crossing over to your left side.

- Tap or bounce your right leg off the ground, bring it back to its original position, and set it on the ground.

- Now switch and take your left leg and move it to the back of your right leg, bounce it off the ground, and then bring it back to its original position.

- You can do this as you move around a room—it may turn out to be a fun activity. Repeat this until satisfied.

NOTE: Keep your torso upright during this exercise.

#: *Lateral Butt Kicks*

To perform lateral butt kicks

- Start by standing tall and in the proper posture.

- Bring the right heel from the ground and raise it as if you want to use it to kick the left butt. As you do this, bring your left hand towards your shoulder as if you are running.

- Switch and do the same with the other side, swinging in motion.

NOTE: To get the most out of this exercise, use the proper posture. Even though the exercise seems simple to perform, doing it the wrong way will not give you the results you desire.

Additionally:

- Your thighs should remain static and fixed in one position as you do the kicks.

- Don't fret if your heel doesn't quite touch your backside as you kick—work on gradually improving your performance.

- Attempt to increase your speed as you go. The faster you go, the faster your heart shall pump, and the more your body shall warm up in readiness for the main exercise.

#: *Jumping*

Jump up and down, front to back and side to side.

#: *Arm Circles and Shoulders*

The steps for this exercise are as follows

- Stand tall with your feet wide apart, and spread your arms out so that they are parallel to the ground.

- Circularly move your arms in small controlled motions as you slowly but gradually make the circles wider until you start to feel your triceps becoming warm.

- Reverse the direction of the circular motion and repeat until satisfied.

#: *Hip Raises*

To perform hip raises:

- Lie on your back, knees slightly bent, and your feet flat on the ground.

- Put your arms to your sides at a 45-degree angle.

- Push out your hips so that your body forms a straight line from the shoulders to the knees. Pause in this position for a few moments.

- Return to the original position.

NOTE: Your trunk and hips should move in unison. The arch in your lower back should remain the same throughout the exercise so that your glutes do the work, not your lower back and hamstrings.

#: *Lunges*

Lunges are a group of activities or movement where you take one of your legs off the ground, take a step either forward, backward, or sideways, and then bend the knee of that leg to form a 90-degree angle while the other leg bends and kneels on the ground.

Then, to complete the move, you retract and go back to your original position.

#: *Hip Rotations*

As the name suggests, these are a group of exercises that engage your hip muscles. You shall encounter such exercise later in this book.

To use hip rotations as a warm-up exercise, hold your waist using both hands, and then rotate your hips in circles.

Stretching Routines

Stretching is not warming up, but it's an essential part of the workout process, especially when it comes to seniors and resistance bands.

Stretching is simple and beneficial to people of all ages, but older adults benefit more from stretching exercises as a way to set the stage for the main workout.

Seniors do not move much during the day. Hence, stretching is vital because it makes the muscles flexible and ready for a workout. A general warm-up should come first, followed by a stretching routine.

The purpose of stretching your muscles is to push the muscle tissues and extend the limits to which they can reach. Stretching will also help you maintain good posture and muscle balance. When your muscle tissues are too tight, it may disrupt force production and exercise performance.

Fundamentally, stretches are either dynamic or static. Dynamic stretches involve repetitive movements, putting the muscles and joints to work. Static stretches, on the other hand, are stagnant. They involve stretching and holding a particular position for a few moments.

Knowing which stretches to engage in, when, and how to use them can help you get the most out of them.

Here are some of the best stretching exercise to engage in before a workout:

#: **Windmill**

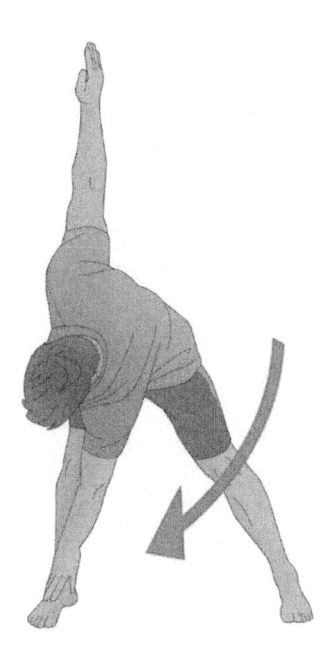

This stretching exercise mainly works on the hamstring, but it has mild effects on the middle and lower back, and calves.

Follow the below steps to perform this stretching exercise.

- Stand with your feet wide open and shoulders apart.

- Spread your arms out to your sides like a pair of wings, so that your body forms the letter "T."

- Stay firmly planted in the ground and unbent as you slowly twist at your waist and move your upper body with your arm progressively going to touch your left foot.

- Return to the original position slowly and repeat the motion in the opposite direction, this time touching the right foot. Repeat this 20 times.

NOTE: You should hold the stretch in position for 20 seconds. Additionally:

- Always keep your legs and arms in a straight position.

- Take deep breaths during the whole time of stretching.

#: Elbow Touch

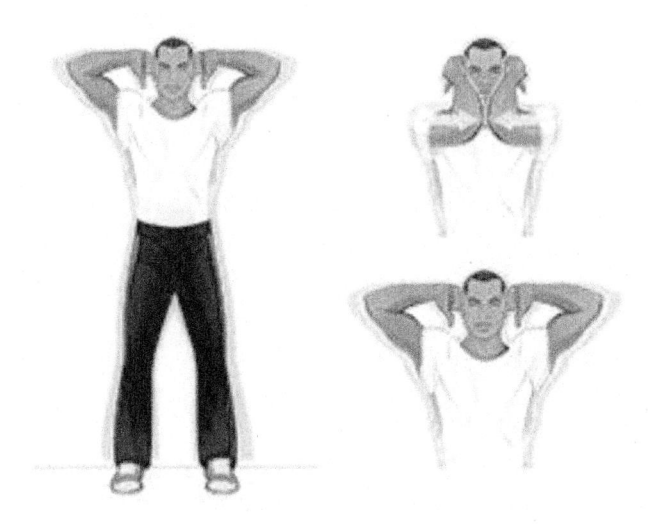

This exercise focuses on the shoulders and neck.

Here's how to perform the elbow touch:

- Stand up straight and place your hands on your shoulders.

- Pull back your elbows and squeeze your shoulder blades together and then hold for a few seconds.

- Bring your elbows back to the original position and then in front of you so they can touch.

#: *Shoulder Box*

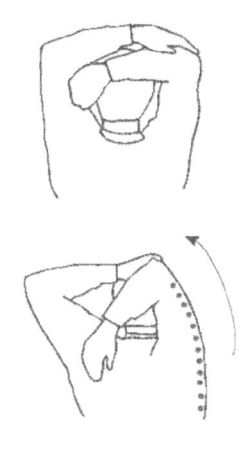

This exercise works out the shoulders and neck muscles. Here's how to perform it:

- Stand up straight in a good posture.

- Inhale deeply through your nose as you lift your shoulders.

- Stick your chest out and pull back your shoulders, then squeeze your shoulder blades.

- Exhaling through your mouth, relax your shoulders, and return to the original position.

#: *Lying Knee to Chest*

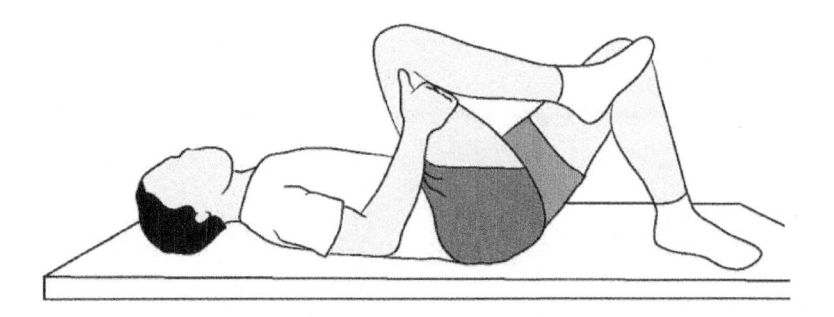

This exercise targets the quadriceps, hamstrings, and calves.

For your safety, begin performing this stretching exercise with only one leg first. If you start feeling comfortable and capable of doing the exercise without any discomfort, upgrade and lift both legs.

If you have a back problem and are uncertain if you should perform this exercise, please seek advice from your healthcare provider.

Here is how to perform this stretching exercise:

- Lie flat on your back—you might need a mat—with your knees bent slightly and your feet firmly resting on the floor. We call this position the supine.

- Slowly and steadily raise one knee enough to hold your lower leg with both hands.

- If you are doing two legs, then bring one leg after the other, not both at the same because raising both legs at the same time a bit tougher. Starting with one leg and following it with the next is a lot safer, especially for seniors.

- As you would do with a single, use your hands to hold your lower legs, just below the knees.

- Slowly pull your knees towards your torso.

- Try to put your legs, pelvis, and lower back at ease as you pull. If done passively, this exercise reaches the muscles in your lower back better.

- Hold for a few moments, and then return to the original position—the supine position.

- Repeat 12 times.

#: *Sit and Reach*

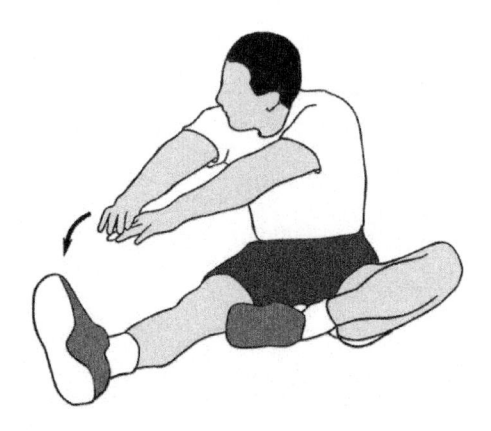

This stretch targets the lower back and hamstrings, and you can use it to test the flexibility of your lower back and hamstring, as well as to determine your susceptibility to pain and injury in the future. Tightness in those two areas in your body can cause muscle pain and stiffness.

To perform this exercise, follow the steps below;

- Take your shoes off and sit on the floor with your legs stretched out, knees unbent.

- Gradually lean forward, hinging from the hips. Keeping your knees straight, stretch out your hand forward and slide them up to your legs as far as you can go, all the way to your toes if you can get there.

- Hold this position for a few moments as you let the stretch do its magic in your back muscles.

- Recoil back to your original position.

- Repeat this several times.

#: Rear Calf Stretch

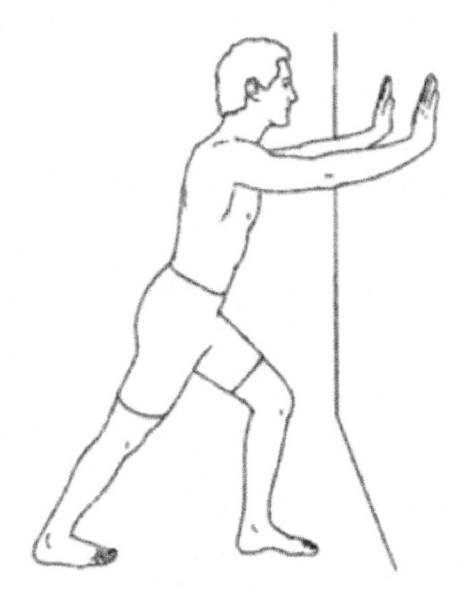

This exercise targets the calf muscles. Here is how to perform it:

- Stand behind a wall or a chair in an upright posture. Place one foot slightly in front of the other and bend the front leg slightly.

- Keep your back knee in a straight position and heel fixed on the ground. Now, slowly lean towards the wall.

- Hold this position for 25 seconds

- Switch legs and repeat the process with the other leg.

- Repeat the routine five times.

Here is a variation of this exercise:

- Stand behind a wall or a chair in an upright posture. Place one foot slightly in front of the other and bend the front leg slightly.

- Bend your back and front knee together but leave your heel fixed on the ground. Now, slowly lean backward away from the wall.

- Hold this position for 25 seconds

- Switch legs and repeat the routine with the other leg.

- Repeat this routine five times

Many physical therapists consider this exercise an effective way to relieve tension in the calves.

#: Gas Pedal

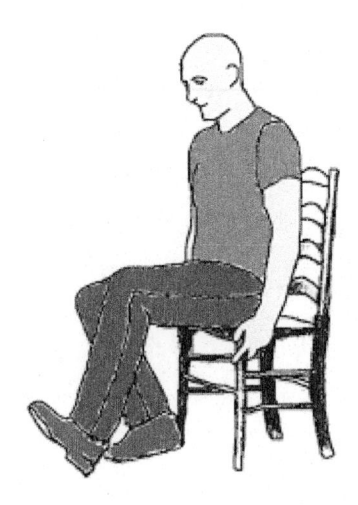

This exercise targets the calf muscles. Here's how to perform it:

- Sit at the edge of a chair, and make sure the chair is stable.

- Lift your right leg slightly, then tilt your foot from the ankle towards your body so that your foot now points to the ceiling.

- Hold this position for a few minutes.

- Push your foot out to point your toes away from your body the same way you would while stepping on the gas pedal when driving.

- Do this for a desirable number of times.

- Switch to the other foot and repeat.

NOTE: Do not force your toe to move in one direction or the other. Be cautious; your calf may cramp as you push your toes forward. Additionally, be careful not to fall off the chair.

#: *Twister*

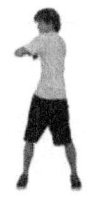

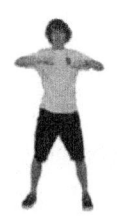

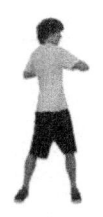

This exercise targets the torso. Here's how to do it:

- Stand straight in good posture.

- Put both your arms across your chest and breathe in slowly and deeply through your nose.

- As you release your breath, twist to your left in a slow and smooth motion.

- Hold this position for as long it feels comfortable, and you can feel your torso muscles stretch.

- Breathe in and return to the original position before you breathe out and twist to the right.

- Hold this position for as long as it is comfortable and feel the torso stretch.

NOTE: If you experience lower back pain, take caution with this exercise.

#: *Side Bend*

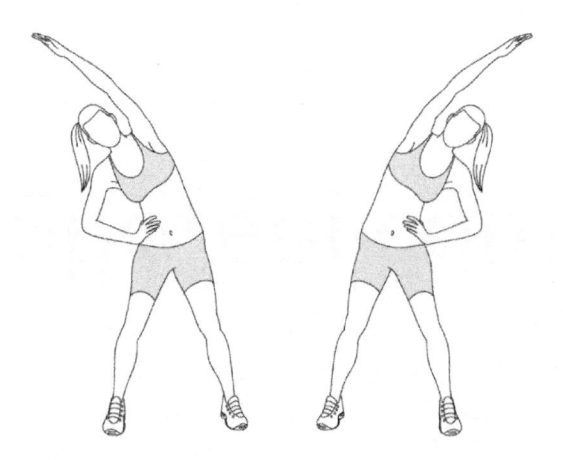

You can perform this either sitting or standing. It targets the muscles between the ribs, the ones that support the ribs

Here's how to perform it:

- Sit in proper posture in a steady chair, placing your feet flat on the floor. For the standing variant, stand with your feet slightly apart.

- Lean forward a little to prevent hunching your shoulders and back.

- Keep your hips, shoulders and ears, shoulders in a straight line.

- Now, raise your right arm over the top of your head to a comfortable height. As you do, breathe in deeply through your nose.

- Breathe out through your mouth slowly as you bend your upper body to the left in a reaching motion, do this smoothly.

- Hold the stretch for a few moments and then switch to the other side of your body, with your left hand raised this time.

- Repeat this a few times.

NOTE: Do not twist to the side as you bend. Additionally:

- Make sure you feel the muscles along the side of your body stretch, from the lower back to your shoulder.

- If your shoulder is stiff, put your hand on top of your head

- If raising your hand causes pain, keep your hands lowered and by your side throughout the stretch.

#: *Rock n Roll*

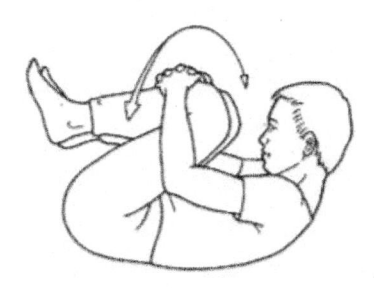

This stretch targets the muscles in the lower back and torso. To perform it, you will need a mat. Here's how to do this routine:

- Lie back and slowly bring both your knees close to your chest.

- Slowly reach out for your knees from under your thigh and interlock your hands in position. You can allow your shoulders to lift off the floor.

- While breathing in through your nose and out through your mouth, gently roll from left to right and then right to the left. Do this in a smooth, rocking motion.

- Enjoy the relaxing feeling and repeat for as long as you can sustain it.

#: *Head Tilt*

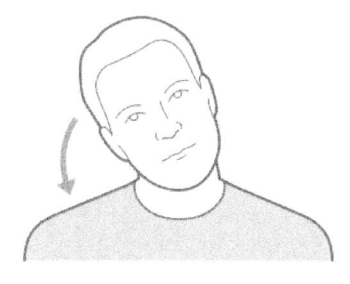

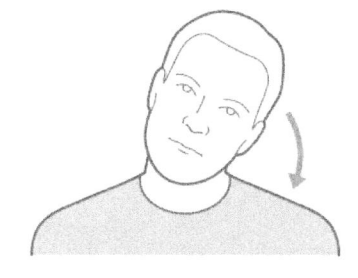

This stretching exercise is relatively easy because it focuses on the neck only. Here are the steps:

- Stand up straight, with proper posture. Breathe in slowly through your nose while gently tilting your head to the left towards your shoulder. Maintain your shoulders in a relaxed and lowered position.

- Breathe out through your lips and hold this position for a few moments.

- Return your head to the original position and repeat but tilt the head going in the opposite direction towards your right shoulder.

- Repeat this as many times as you can.

NOTE: Do not be rough or vigorous.

#: *Tennis Watcher*

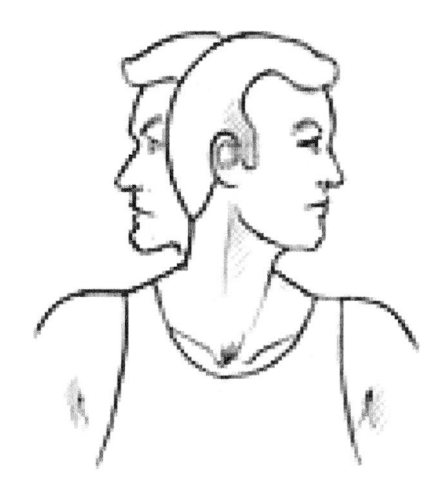

Judging from the name, you can probably guess what this stretching exercise looks like: periodically looking to your left and right, which, if you have been to a tennis match, you understand. This exercise works on the neck muscles. Here is how to do it:

- Stand up straight. Breathe in slowly through the nose and as you do this, look as far to your left as you can without feeling any discomfort.

- Breathe out through your mouth and hold this position for a few moments, feeling your muscles stretch.

- Now, breathe in gently through your mouth and switch to looking to the right, slowly.

- Breathe out through your mouth and hold your position.

- Repeat this as many times as desired.

NOTE: Remember to be gentle.

#: *Shoulder Box*

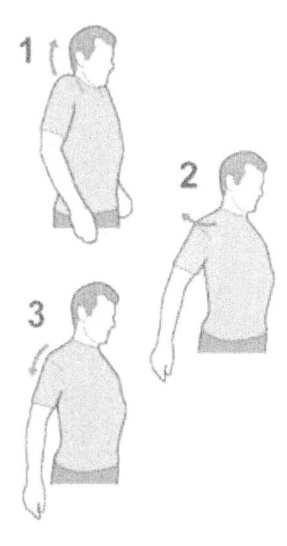

Here is how to perform this stretch that works out the Trapezius:

- Stand up straight and breathe in through your nose as you slowly lift your shoulders.

- Pull your shoulders back and your shoulder blades together and down.

- Breathe out through your mouth, relax your shoulders, and return to the original position.

- Repeat as many times as desired.

Having looked at how to warm up and stretch, we can move on and discuss effective resistance band workouts for seniors, but before we do, let's discuss some measures you should observe:

Section 3

Resistance Band Workout Guidelines

Before you start exercising with resistance bands, you need to know and observe a few essential things, the most important of which are:

#: *Mind the pain*

Everyone can use resistance bands. However, if you suffer from an existing medical condition such as a severe joint problem, start performing the exercises without the bands and do it for two weeks. Once your muscles have accustomed to the movements, you can gradually introduce the bands in your workouts.

Once you can perform routines without an increase in pain, it's time to incorporate the bands in your exercises fully. The rule of thumb is that if you experience pain two hours after working out, what you are doing is not suitable for you.

#: *Choose your band wisely*

Choosing a band that has the correct resistance level is crucial.

Unfortunately, it is common for many people to use the same resistance band for all exercises. Although doing this is fine and can produce the desired results, using a lighter band for specific exercises like triceps exercises and then a tougher band for your much stronger muscles like the chest and legs is ideal and yields better results.

#: *Maintain Good Posture*

Good posture is a prerequisite for a good and safe training session. Always sit on your sitting bones, not your tail bone. If you sit on your tail bone, it means you are slouching, with your spine bent, which can cause back pain. Make sure you always sit tall: don't slouch!

When standing during a workout session, stand with your spine in a proper neutral posture. From the side view, your ears should look aligned with your shoulders.

Your shoulders should be over your hips, and your hips over the ankles. Your weight should feel equally distributed between your two feet, and your knees bent slightly. Your hips should rest in their natural and relaxed position, neither tilted upwards nor downwards. Maintain your chest high and your back straight at all times.

Below are ten tips for a successful and effective workout. We have mentioned some in other chapters, but for reinforcement purposes, they are worth listing here in again so that you can have them in one place:

1. Always prepare your body for resistance training by performing a full-body warm-up. Never skimp on this.

2. Make sure you are in top-notch health before you begin exercising. If you are not sure of what you can or cannot do in these exercises, please consult your physician first.

3. Remember to do the movements of the exercises while in proper posture and with sound biomechanics. Do not sacrifice form for shoddy repetitions.

4. Never hold your breath while working out. Good breathing patterns go well with workouts, so get that air circulating in your lungs. Holding your breath will cause high blood pressure and dizziness. Exhale when performing the most challenging parts and inhale as you recoil back to the original or resting position.

5. Listening to your body is another vital thing to consider. A little soreness in the muscles after exercise is normal and okay, but when an exercise increases a persistent pain, consider that a red flag. In such a scenario, you should stop engaging in that exercise. Always pay attention to how your body responds to every workout routine.

6. To get the desired outcome, create a regular workout routine. Ideally, you should partake in resistance band training two or three times a week.

7. Keep training, but don't kill yourself while at it. Don't bite off more than you can chew and don't strain. It is okay to take it slow occasionally. The important thing is to create a consistent workout routine.

8. Get into the habit of checking the condition of your resistance band, even during training, for wear and tear.

9. Perform the movements slowly and with great control. Do not allow the band to slip off your hand and snapback; this can cause injury. Control the band, do not let it control you!

10. Do the exercise using a full range of motion.

Keeping these tips in mind, let's start discussing the most effective resistance band workouts:

Section 4

Resistance Band Workout Exercises For Seniors

Upper Body Exercises

These exercises focus on the upper body:

#: One Arm Triceps Extension

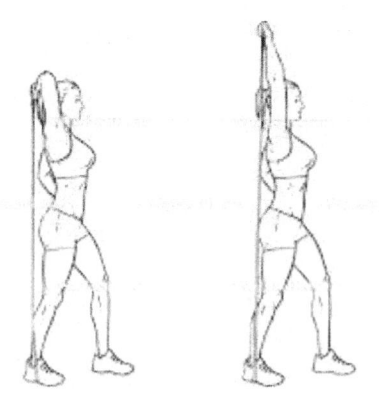

Here's how to perform the one arm tricep extension:

- Stand upright, putting your right foot slightly in front of your left foot, in a manner that looks like a staggered stance.

- Use your left foot to stand on one end of the resistance band. Now, using your right hand, grab the other end of your resistance band and position it behind your neck; the right elbow should be pointing up. That is your starting position.

- Move your right hand upwards until the elbow is straight.

- Put it down slowly to the original position.

- Perform several repetitions with your right arm, and then switch sides to the left side of your body, and repeat for a desired number of repetitions.

#: *Two Arm Triceps Extensions*

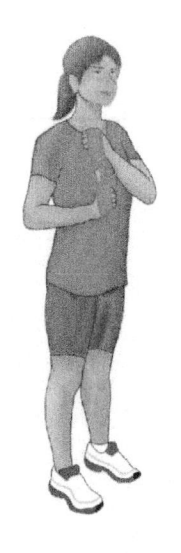

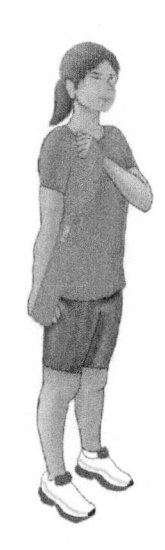

- Take one end of the band with your left hand and place it against your collar bone.

- Grab the other end with your right hand then position it at chest level.

- While maintaining your right elbow positioned in and down, stretch your right arm at full stretch.

- At all times during these movements, make sure that your left hand remains at a braced position at your mid-back.

#: Horizontal Arm Extensions

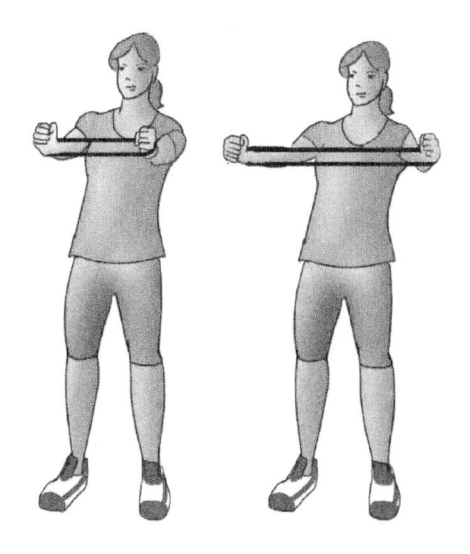

- Stand up tall in good posture, making sure to maintain a straight back. Put your hands inside the resistance band as if to cuff yourself with them, your wrists holding both ends.

- Stretch your hands out in front of your chest.

- Pull your hands apart to stretch the resistance band, making sure that as you do this, you keep your hands slightly bent. Ensure that your hands are moving in a straight line parallel to the ground.

- When you reach the maximum length to which you can stretch your arms, Pause for a moment, recoil to the original position, and then repeat for the desired number of times.

#: *Vertical Arm Extensions*

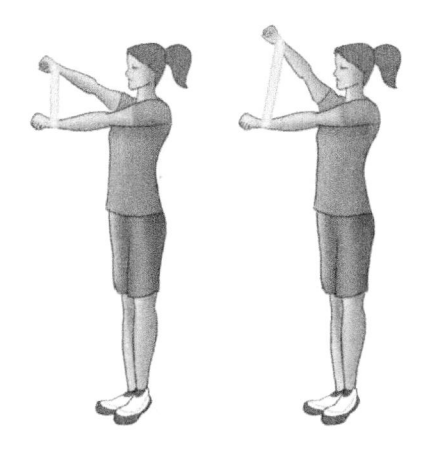

This exercise is similar to the horizontal arm extension, but as the name suggests, in this case, the arms are moving along a vertical plane.

- Stand up tall in good posture and maintain a straight back. Put your hands inside the resistance band as if to cuff yourself with them, your wrists holding both ends.

- Stretch your hands out in front of your chest. One hand should be at the level of your head, the other in front of your stomach.

- Pull your hands apart to stretch the resistance band. Ensure that your hands are moving in a straight line perpendicular to the ground.

- When you reach the maximum length you can stretch your arms, pause for a moment, then recoil back to the original position, and repeat for the desired number of repetitions.

#: Rear Arm Extensions

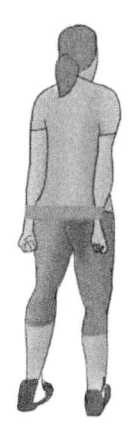

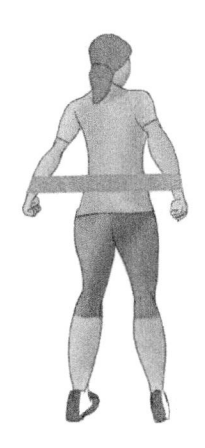

- Stand tall with your feet slightly apart. Put your hands behind your back. Then, place the resistance band around your wrists so that it looks like a handcuff around your hands.

- Now start pushing your hands apart to stretch the resistance band; keep your hands slightly bent as you do this. Make sure your hands are moving in a straight line horizontal to the ground.

- When you reach the maximum length to which you can stretch your arms, pause for a moment.

- Recoil back to the original position then repeat for the desired number of reps.

#: Upright Row

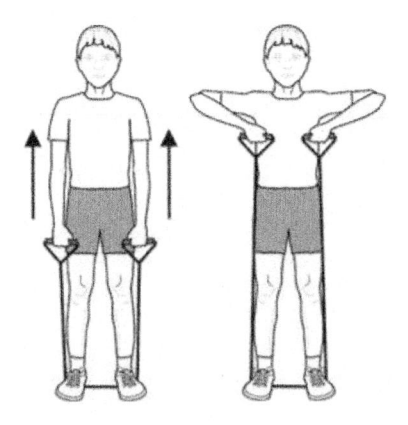

- Step on your resistance band with both feet.

- Take one end of the band and crisscross it with the other end so that it forms an "X" in front of you.

- With a tight grip, pull both ends with your hands all the way to shoulder level, spreading your hands out like wings on your sides as you pull the resistance band.

- Slowly lower your hands down to the starting position.

- Repeat this as many times as you desire.

#: *Bicep Curl*

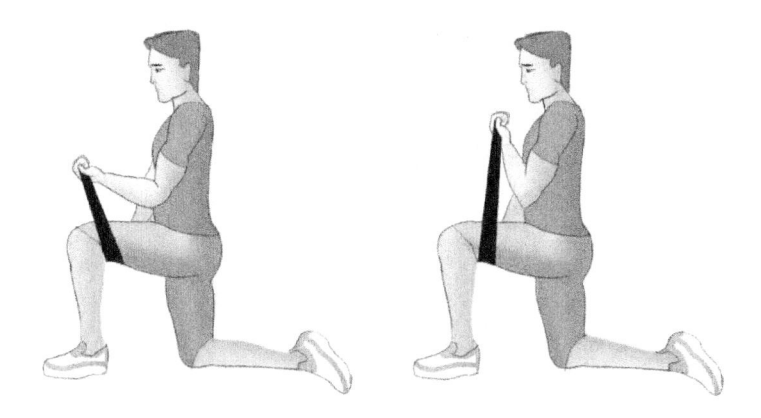

- Put your left leg into the circle of the resistance band and drive it up to the knee.

- Kneel on the other knee and, with a firm grip, hold the resistance band locked in your knee.

- Slowly pull the band with your hand to your chest in a curly move—hence the name—keeping your elbow in a fixed position.

- When you reach the peak, pause for a moment, and then slowly retract back to the original position

#: Lunge with Biceps Curl

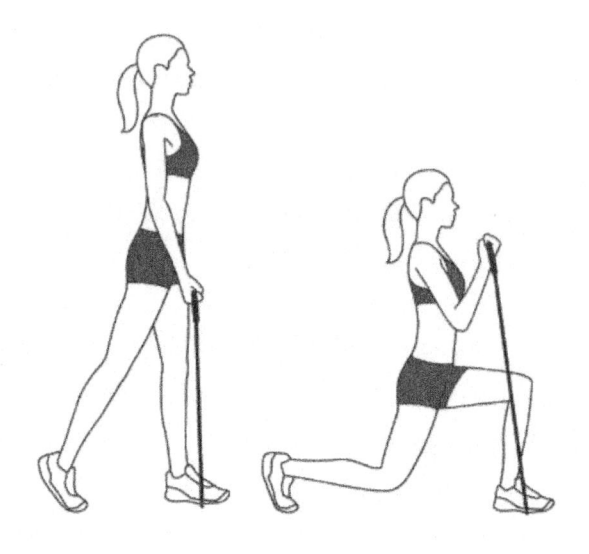

- Put your left foot inside the resistance band and then grab the other end with your right hand.

- For balance, put your right leg slightly behind.

- Slowly bend your left knee as you slide your right leg further back to get into a lunge position as if you are about to propose.

- As you go up and down, use your left hand for support.

- As you are making these movements, you will pull the resistance band to do the bicep curl.

- Come back up slowly, and repeat this several times before switching to the other foot and hand.

#: Bent-Over Row

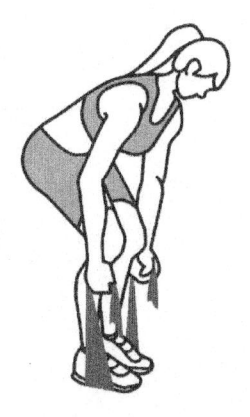

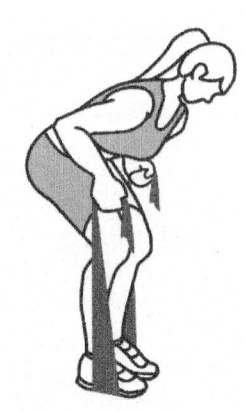

- Start by standing while both feet are placed on the resistance band making sure that the feet are placed hip-width apart.

- Then grab one end of the resitance band in each hand on the sides making sure that your palms are facing towards each other.

- Next, slightly bend your knees then hinge about 30 degrees forward on the hips. As you do that, be sure to ensure that your arms are straight, the back is flat and the hands are nicely tacked under the shoulders.

- Then bend the elbows to allow you to pull the band towards the chest. Be sure to straighten the arms and then lower the hands back to your starting position.

- This makes one rep.
- Perform as many reps are you can.

Lower Body Exercises

#: *Bridge Thrusts*

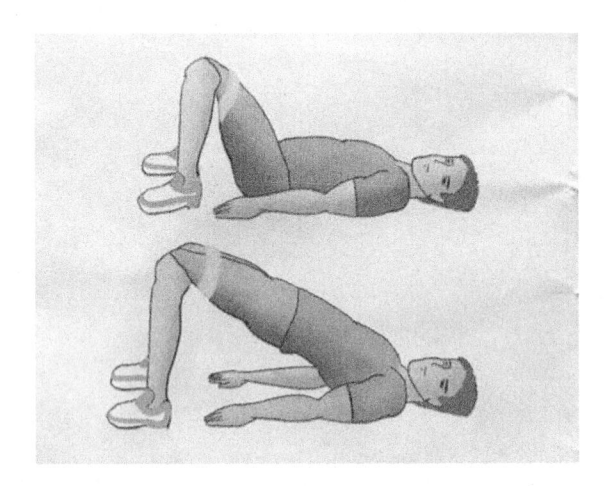

- Insert both legs inside the circle of the resistance band. Pull the band to just above the knees where your thighs begin.

- Lie on your back with your knees slightly bent

- Thrust your hips upwards and into the air while firmly fixing your hands on the ground.

- Pause in this position for a few moments.

- Retract to the original position slowly.

#: Side Step Squats

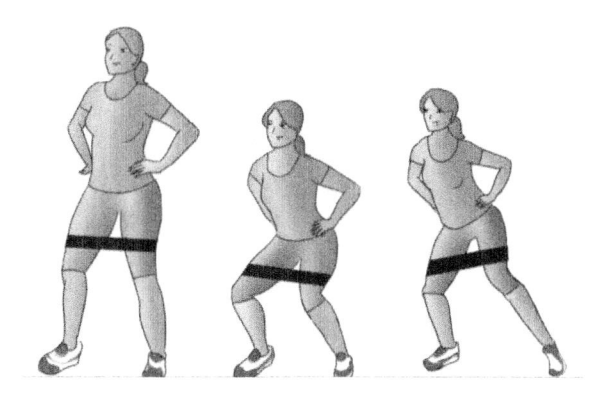

- Place your legs inside the loop of the resistance band, just above your knees.

- Stand in the correct posture, with your legs slightly apart.

- Push your right leg out to your side while simultaneously going down for a slight squat.

- Pause in the squat position for a moment, then return to the original position.

#: Hug-the-World Plié

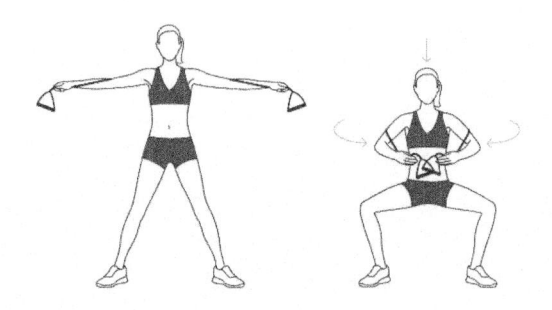

- Stand tall with your back straight and feet slightly apart, feet looking away from each other.

- Stretch your hands out straight.

- Take the resistance band and put it on top of your shoulder, running from one hand to the other as you hold onto each end.

- Bring your hands together as if you want to hug the air and simultaneously go down as if to squat, but stop when you reach the level where your thighs are parallel to the ground. You are going to feel the resistance pull in your hands.

- Open up your hug as you go back to the original position

- Do this several times

#: *Lying Hip Abductions*

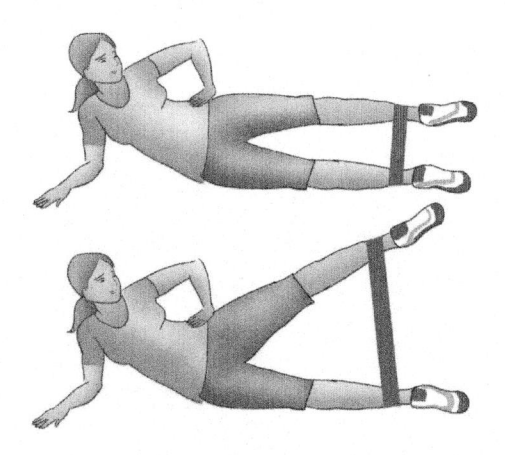

- Take the resistance band and put it around your legs just above the ankles

- Lie on the ground on your right side, put your right elbow on the ground for support so that you slightly raise your upper body. Pile your left leg on top of the right one.

- Pull your left leg away from the right one upwards, stretching the resistance band as you do this.

- When you reach the peak of your stretch, pause in that position for a moment.

- Retract and go back to your original position.

- When finished, switch and do the left side also.

#: Squat with Overhead Press

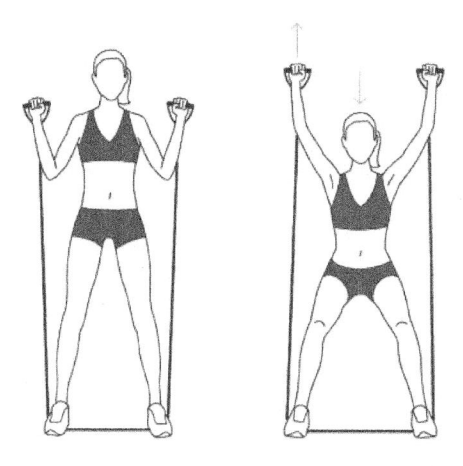

- Stand tall with both your feet stepping on the resistance band.

- While using each of your hands to hold each end of the resistance band, pull the resistance band as high as you can with your hands facing upwards; this is the start position.

- Push your hands into the sky against the force of the band while simultaneously going down, slightly bending your knees. Repeat for a desired number of reps.

#: *Lying Leg Raises*

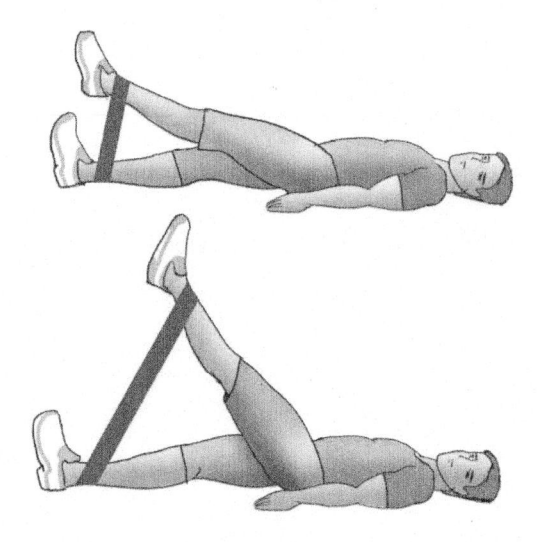

Lying leg raises are similar to the lying hip abductions exercise in the sense that the resistance band remains around your legs.

- Lie on the ground, facing the ceiling, with the resistance band around your ankles.

- Keep your hands fixed to the ground.

- Pull one leg away from the other, going upwards towards the ceiling as far as you can. When you reach the furthest stretch point, pause for a few moments.

- Bring your leg down to its original position and do the exercise with your other leg.

- Keep up this motion—as if you are walking in the air—and repeat until you hit your reps target.

#: Standing Hip Abductions

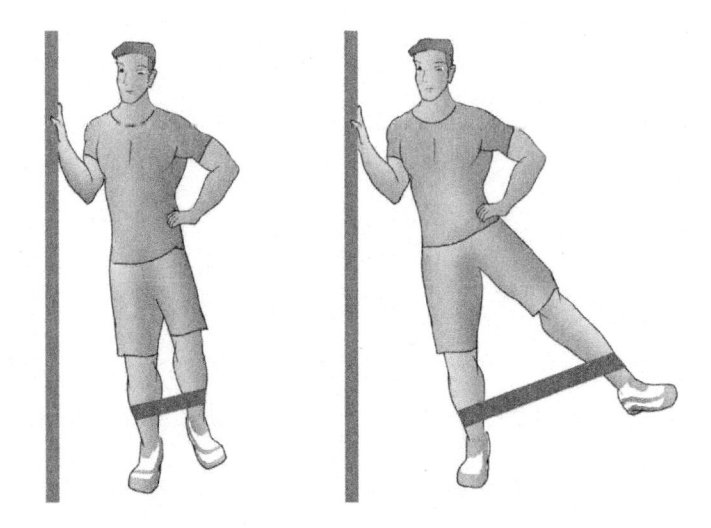

Standing hip abductions are similar to the lying hip abductions; however, in this case, you perform the exercise from a standing up position.

- Put the resistance band around your legs and pull them up to ankle-level.

- Find a wall for support and hold on to it with your right hand, then pull your left leg away from your right one so that you stretch the resistance band.

- Stretch to your furthest possible point and when you get to that point, pause for a moment.

- Slowly return your leg to its original position and then repeat.

- When satisfied, switch to holding the wall with your left hand and then pull out your right leg.

Abdominal Exercises

#: Oblique Overhead Extension

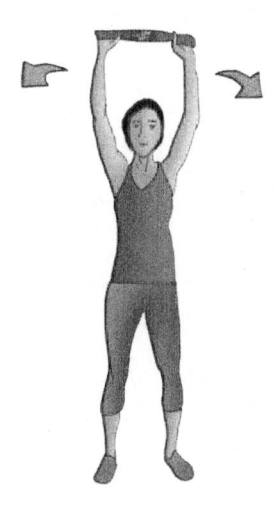

- Grab your resistance band from both ends and raise it above your head, making sure to stand tall and in good posture, your back straight and legs slightly apart.

- Slowly pull your hands apart, stretching the bands as far as you can go.

- When you reach the farthest end, pause for a moment, and hold your position.

- Return slowly to the original position. Repeat this movement several times until satisfied.

#: *Bicycles*

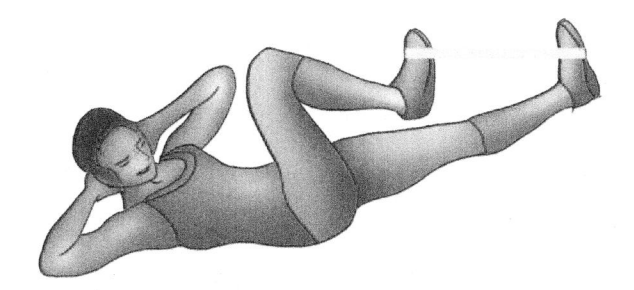

- Place the resistance band around your ankles and lie down on the ground facing the ceiling. With your hands at the back of your head and your back fixed on the ground, raise both feet into the air.

- Pull your right knee in close to your chest while at the same stretching and pushing your left elbow up until it touches your knee. Don't worry if you do not actually make contact with your knee.

- Return to the resting position and then alternate to bring your left knee to your chest while you straighten your right leg, and at the same time, push your right elbow to touch your left knee.

#: Ab Crunch with Rotation

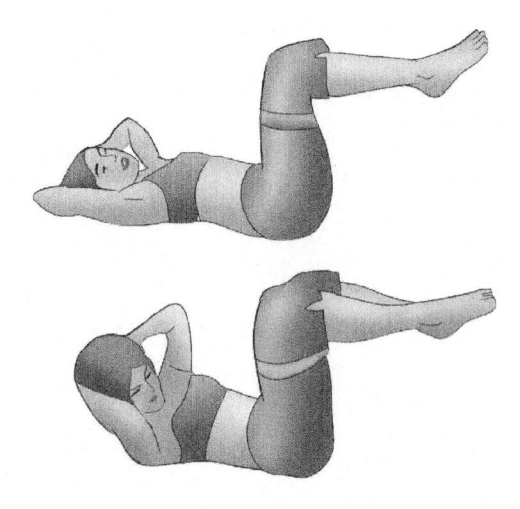

- Lie flat on the ground, facing the ceiling with the loop of your resistance band inside your two legs above the thighs.

- Raise your legs in the air and place your hand at the back of your head. Remember to keep the resistance band above your thighs.

- Lift your head and bring your opposite knee towards your head. At the same time, spread your thighs apart to stretch the band.

- As you come out of this position and back into the resting position, breath out through your mouth.

- Repeat this in the opposite direction and continue with the routine until you feel satisfied.

Seated Concentration Curl

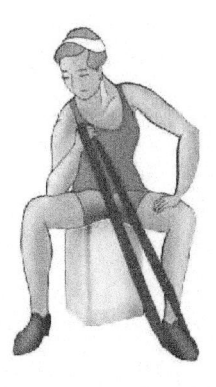

- Find a position on which to sit and place one of the ends of the resistance band under your left foot.

- Next, use your right hand to grab the other end of the resistance band. Rest your right elbow on your right thigh, and rest your other hand on your left thigh for balance.

- Pull the resistance band to your chest, making a curve. When you reach your chest, take a pause, and then return to the original position.

- Repeat this, and when satisfied, switch, and do the exercise with the opposite side of your body.

#: Triceps Extension

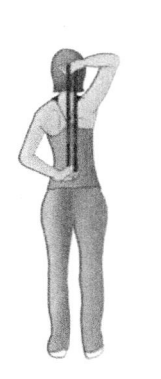

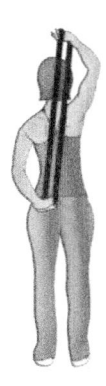

- Stand tall with your legs slightly apart and in a comfortable and stable position.

- Grasp one end of the resistance band in your right hand and throw it to your back so that the other end of the band is hanging loose toward your butt.

- Reach out for the loose end of the band behind you with your left hand and grab it.

- Pull the band with your right hand up above your head in a straight line while keeping the left hand stationary by your lower back

- Repeat this motion several times and then switch hands.

Chest Exercises

#: Incline Chest Press

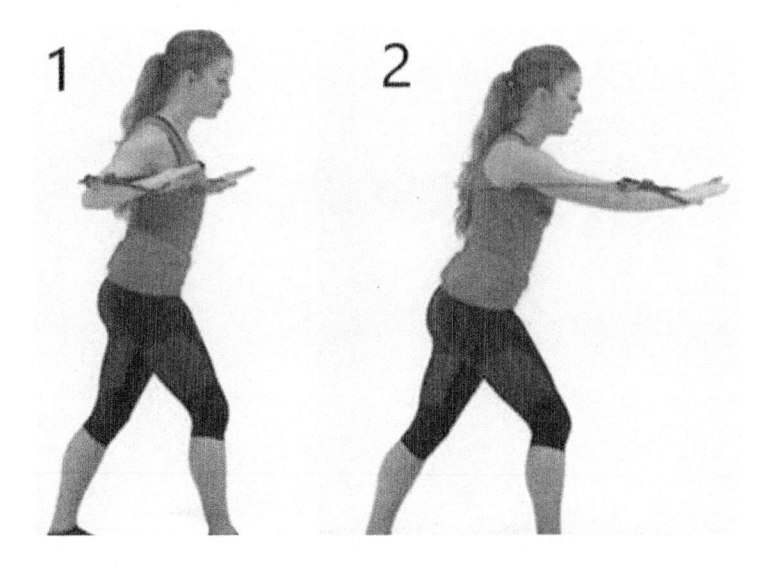

You can perform this exercise from a sitting or standing position:

- Run the resistance band behind your back, just under your armpit, with each end of the band held in your hands to make the starting position.

- Keep your wrists straight and unbent as you hold the band and push out straight in front of you, stretching the band until your hands are straight and out, pointing to the front.

- Slowly return to the starting position.
- Repeat this several times.

Shoulder Exercises

#: *Frontal Raise*

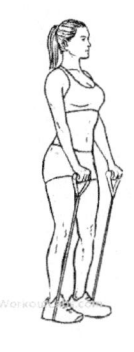

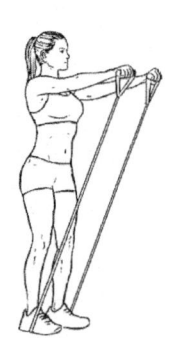

- Sit or stand on the resistance band and hold each end in each hand.

- Your hands should rest on the front part of your thighs.

- Adjust the resistance band for the desired resistance.

- Keeping your hands and wrists straight, pull the band upwards, bringing your hands vertically in front of you but not past your shoulder height.

- Hold this position for a few moments, then slowly lower your hands to the original starting position.

- Repeat this several times

You can do this with one hand at a time, alternating between one hand and the other.

#: Shoulder Press

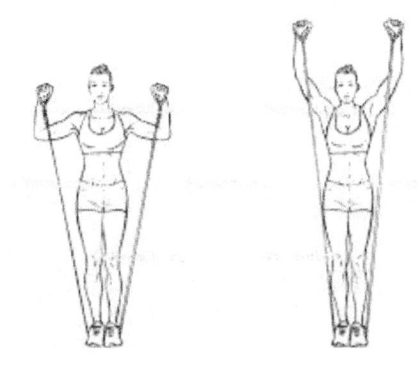

NOTE: If you have a history of shoulder-related issues, avoid this exercise.

- Step on the resistance band in the middle with both of your legs while standing. Make sure your legs are close together. With your left hand, grab the left side, and with your right hand grab the left.

- Rise up to stand straight while still holding the ends of the bands. Pull the resistance and position your hands to face upwards so as to make a 90- degree angle at your eblow joints. This is the starting point.

- Push your hands over and above your head until your hands are completely straight and pose for a moment in this position.

- Slowly return back to the starting position.

- Repeat this several times.

You can also perform this exercise with one arm at a time, alternating between the hands.

#: *Lateral Arm Raise*

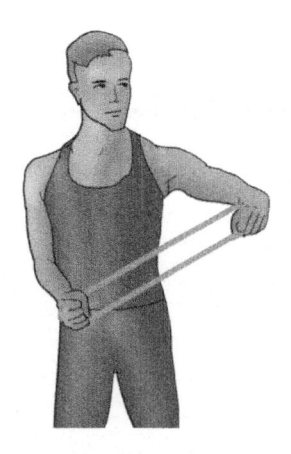

- Stand tall and stable, your feet grounded. Make sure your hands have a firm grip on both ends of the resistance band.

- Lift both your hand up to your chest, and with your right hand, stretch out as if to punch the air in front of you. Keep your left hand fixed and close to your chest.

- Stretch the band to the farthest possible point and then hold that position for a few moments.

- Return your right hand to your chest and then alternate and push out your left hand while your right hand remains fixed to that resistance force on the right hand.

#: Crunch with Lat Pull-Down

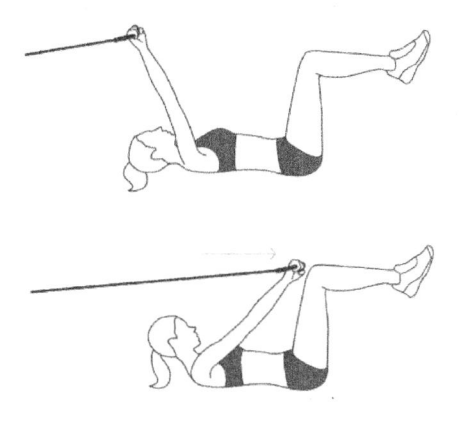

- Find a stable and stationary structure and loop the resistance band around it.

- Hold the ends of the resistance band in your hands, each hand holding an end.

- Lie down on your back with your knee bent and leg raised off the ground to form a 90-degree angle at your knee.

- Pull the band from where you are lying against its resistance force towards your knees, making sure your hands remain straight at all times.

Back Exercises

#: Lat Pull-down

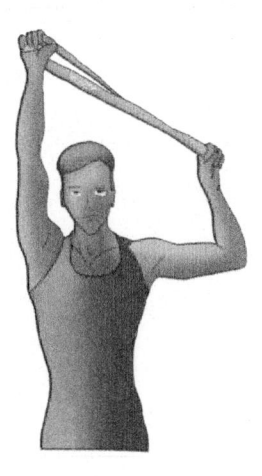

- Find some balance and stand with your legs slightly apart. Hold the resistance band at both ends and raise it above your head.

- Pull both ends of the resistance band down and apart at the same time so that a lot of the force you use comes from your back, not your arms.

- When you achieve the maximum stretch for the band, pause for a moment and then return to the original position.

- Repeat this sequence several times.

#: *Seated Rowing*

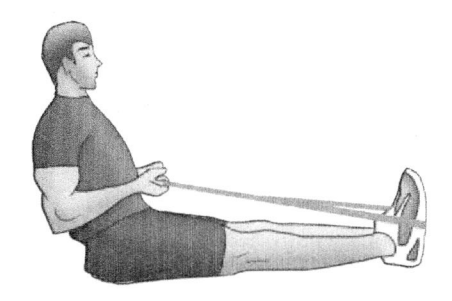

- Sit on the ground with your legs stretched in front of you. Take the resistance band and fix it below your feet—as if you are stepping on it. Hold the other end in both hands.

- Now pull the band from your feet to a full stretch as you tilt your body backward so that you make a rowing movement.

- Slowly retract to the original position and do the movement again.

- Repeat until you feel satisfied.

Thigh Exercises

#: Band Squats

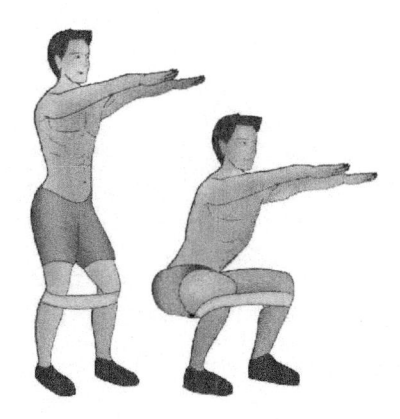

- Stand with your legs slightly apart, making sure you are looking forward and in front of you. Pull the resistance band loop around your thigh area.

- Stretch both hands out so that they are sticking out in midair and parallel to the ground.

- Move down slowly and gently to a squatting position until your thighs reach a horizontal plane, and then hold that position for a few moments.

- Return to your original position slowly and steadily.

- Repeat this movement for the amount of desired reps.

#: Seated Leg Extensions

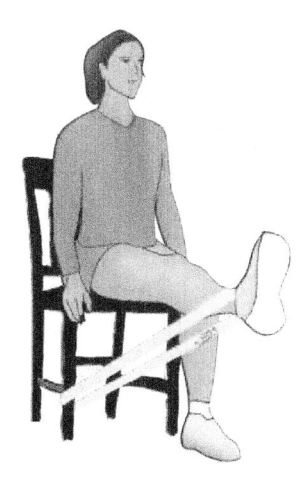

- Find a steady chair and fix one end of the resistance band around the foot of the chair in a way that ensures it won't budge. Put the other end of the band around your right ankle.

- Slowly kick out your right leg to stretch the resistance band. When you reach the peak of the stretch, hold that position for a few moments.

- Return the right leg to its original position slowly and repeat the movement several times.

- When you complete your desired number of reps, switch and give the left leg some action too.

#: *Clamshell*

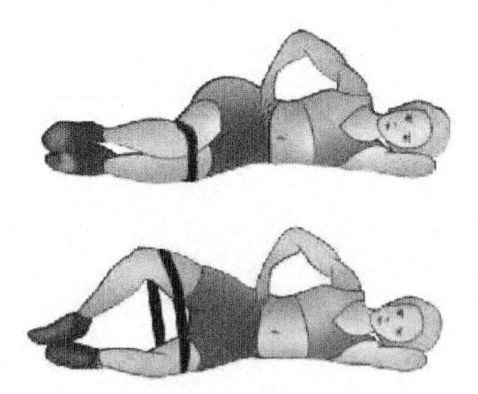

- Lie on the ground on your right side, with your hand under your head to act as a headrest. Put the resistance band loop around your legs and bring it up to your thighs, just above the knees.

- Use your left hand to hold your waist for balance.

- Keep your legs together and bent to form a 90-degree angle.

- While your feet remain touching and locked together, pull your knees apart from each other to stretch the resistance band. When you reach the peak, hold the position for a few seconds.

- Return to the original position slowly and steadily.

- Repeat this several times, and once you've hit your rep goal, switch and repeat the exercise with the other leg.

Glute and Hip Flexor Exercises

#: *Thigh Thrusts*

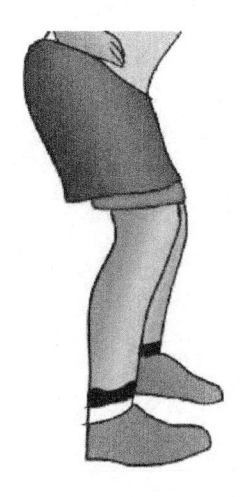

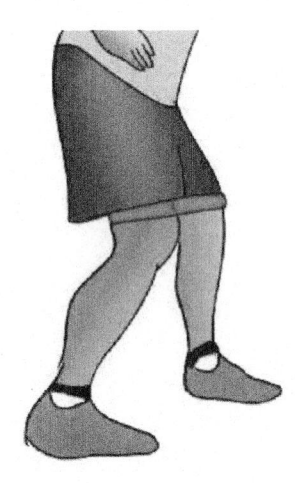

- Place your legs inside the loop of the resistance band, slightly above your knee in your thigh area.

- Take three steps forward and then three steps backward as you resist the force applied by the resistance band.

- Repeat the exercise and keep pressing against the force of the resistance band.

#: *Lateral Walk*

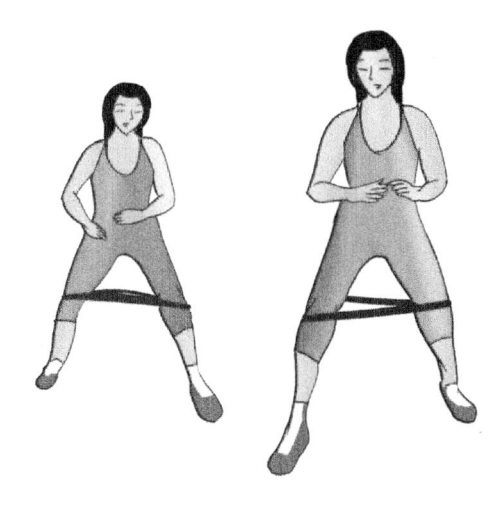

This exercise differs slightly from the thigh thrusts exercise above.

- Pull the resistance band around your knees, keeping your legs spread wide.

- Put one leg forward, and the other back like a boxer would stand in the ring. Make sure your back is straight.

- Move the leg behind forward and in front of the other one. That should make a big step to the right to give the resistance band a nice and clean stretch. Repeat the process with the leg that is now behind to take another step.

- Keep doing this several times

#: *Standing Hip Flexion*

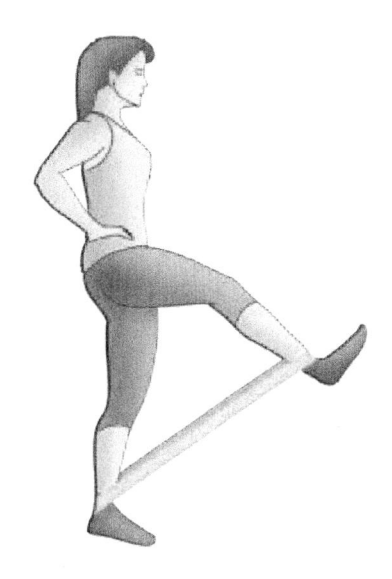

- Stand tall, holding your waist for support, with your legs slightly apart, and the resistance band looped around your ankles.

- Keep one leg straight and firmly fixed on the ground as you push out one leg forward to stretch the resistance.

- When you've stretched to the furthest point you can, hold for a few seconds and then slowly bring it down to its resting position on the ground.

- Do several reps and then alternate and repeat the procedure with the other leg as well.

#: Single-Leg Loop Bridge

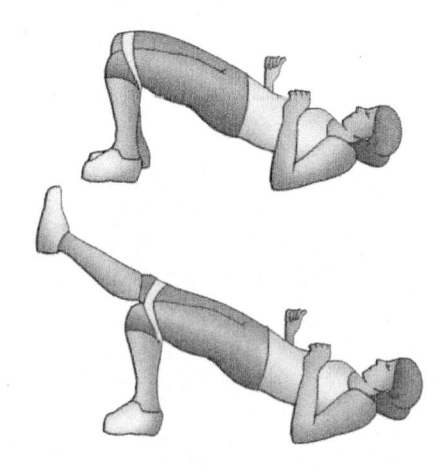

- Put the resistance band around your legs and pull it up to your thighs, and then lie flat on your back, looking up at the ceiling.

- Bend your knees so that your feet are stepping on the ground. Then, raise the trunk of your body so that you make a straight line from your knee to your neck.

- Keep your back in a straight position. While in this position, take one foot off the ground and raise it in the air until it's parallel to your spine. At the same time, pull your legs apart as you go against the force of the band.

- Pause and hold this position for a few moments before slowly bringing your foot back to its resting position on the ground.

- Switch and do the same with the other foot and repeat until you achieve your reps goal.

#: Side Lunge with Side Raise

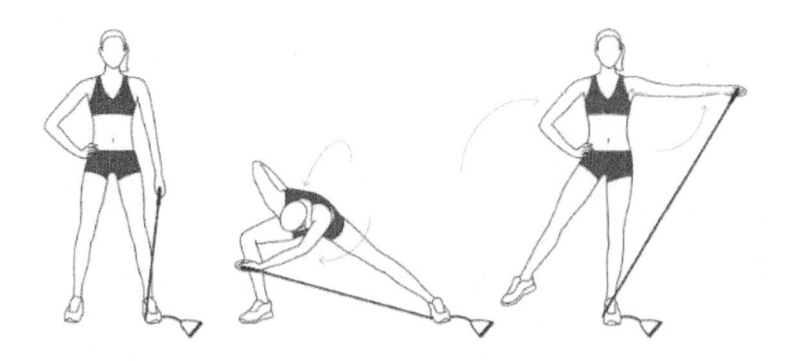

- Stand tall with your feet slightly wide apart, with your left foot stepping on one end of the resistance band.

- Hold the other end of the band firmly in your left hand and put your right hand on your waist. That is your starting position.

- Take your right foot off the ground and step outside to your right and into a lunge.

- As you do this, swing your left hand to the right in the direction of the right foot and bend forward as if you're taking a bow.

- To return to the original position, push out your right foot to propel you back up to the standing position. Repeat this several times

- Switch and perform this with the other side of your body.

Calf Exercise

#: Seated Calf Press

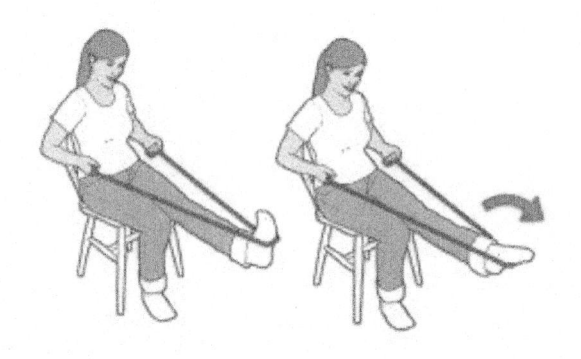

- Sit on a chair with your back straight. Put the resistance band under your left foot and hold each end in each of your hands.

- As you hold the resistance band, extend your leg out straight, stretching the band in the process.

- Tilt your foot forward by pointing your toes out in front. Bring your foot back and repeat this several times

- Switch and do the exercise with your right leg as well.

Section 5

Cooling Down

Essentially, cooling down, which is an essential part of your workout routine, involves continuing to do the exercises for a few more minutes, albeit at a slower rate and reduced intensity.

Cooling down reduces the strain your muscles might otherwise experience when you shift from a warm-up state to a cold state too. Cooling down operates on the precepts that make warming up necessary. Cooling down helps prevent fatigue and is also relaxing.

The following six exercises that can help your muscles and body cool down. Perform these exercises slower and with lesser intensity than you did the resistance band exercises.

#: Seated Forward Bend

- Sit on the ground with your legs stacked together and stretched in front of you.

- Keep your hands touching the ground and by the sides of your waist.

- Now bend forward from the waist to touch your toes with your hand, and bow your head deep to touch your knees.

- Raise your head back and go to the original position.

- Repeat at an even slower pace.

#: *Standing Forward Bend*

- Stand tall on your feet.
- Bend and bow to touch your toes.
- Repeat.

#: *Knee to Chest Pose*

- Lie flat on your back and raise one leg to your chest.

- As your leg reaches the chest, hold it with both hands and press it on your chest, then release it back to the ground.

- Do the same with the other leg.

- Keep this movement going steadily but slowly.

#: Child's Pose

- Place your hands and feet on the ground and your waist in the air. Your head should face down.

- Bring your knees down to a kneeling position and then proceed to sit on your legs and finally resting your chest on your thighs, your hands still in position, holding the ground. At this point, rest your forehead on the ground.

- Rise above again and repeat

- Keep up the rhythm

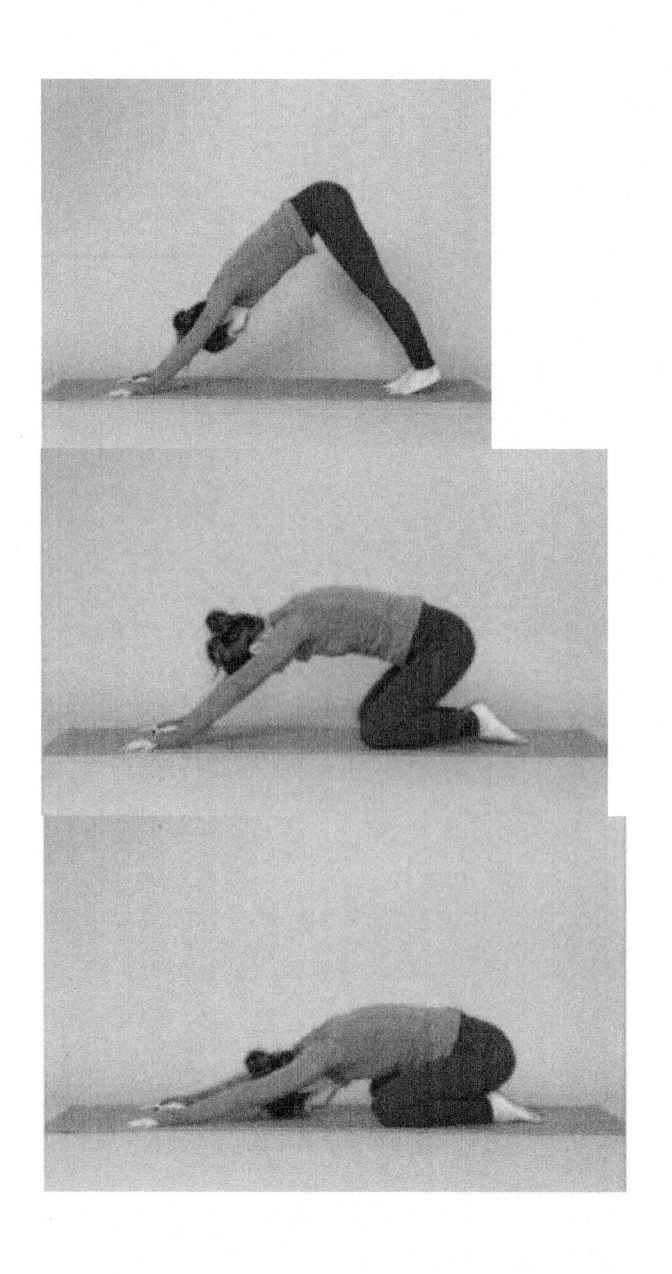

#: *Legs Up the Wall Pose*

- Lie down next to a wall and swing your legs up along the wall.

- Place your hands on your stomach and hold this pose for however long you want.

#: *Corpse Pose*

- Lie on your back, facing the ceiling.

- Roll both hands on the ground so that your palms open and close in a repetitive motion

- Roll your legs as well.

- Relax as you feel your muscles ease into a state of cool down.

Section 6

Resistance Band Workout Programs

This section features several training programs designed for seniors with a wide range of needs, depending on prevailing health situations or target muscles.

As mentioned earlier, as you exercise, do not sacrifice quality for quantity. Do not compromise form so that you can finish a workout routine fast. Instead, make sure you are working your joints out through the full range of motion, which means you should do each exercise seamlessly and with deliberateness.

Additionally, as a beginner, choose a band whose resistance level allows you to do one set of eight repetitions for twelve days. After 12 days, add an extra set of eight reps to your routine. For the best form, do one set, take a 40-second rest, and then proceed to the next set.

This section shall discuss several workout programs designed for people at different levels of fitness.

After going through them, you may want to design a resistance band training program that suits you precisely. When it comes to that:

What to Keep In Mind When Designing a Personal Resistance Band Training Program

If you do decide to create a personal resistance band training program, be sure to make it fun and focused on helping improve your fitness and the functionality of your muscles and joints.

Be careful not to fall into the trap of creating a program that overworks certain muscles more than it does others. If you do this, it will only lead to injury and postural imbalance.

Working on a muscle or muscle group too much can have adverse effects on your health; on the other hand, exercising a muscle too little will not yield the results you seek. For this reason, it is good practice to change your program every three months to adopt a new one.

To create a training program that caters to your specific needs, and that helps develop your entire body evenly, first determine your particular health status and work out aims and objectives. Seek your doctor's advice so that you can learn what you can do and what you should avoid

Each workout program should typically have twelve exercises or less. These selected exercises should cater to all your body's major muscles and muscle groups. If you want to do more sets, remember to reduce the number of exercises.

Additionally, consider your daily activities. If, for example, you jog every morning, you should have a training program that doesn't dwell too much on the muscles responsible for jogging so that you don't risk overworking that set of muscles.

Having discussed what you should keep in mind when creating as personalized resistance band workout, here now are various workout programs for different levels:

Beginner's Workout Program

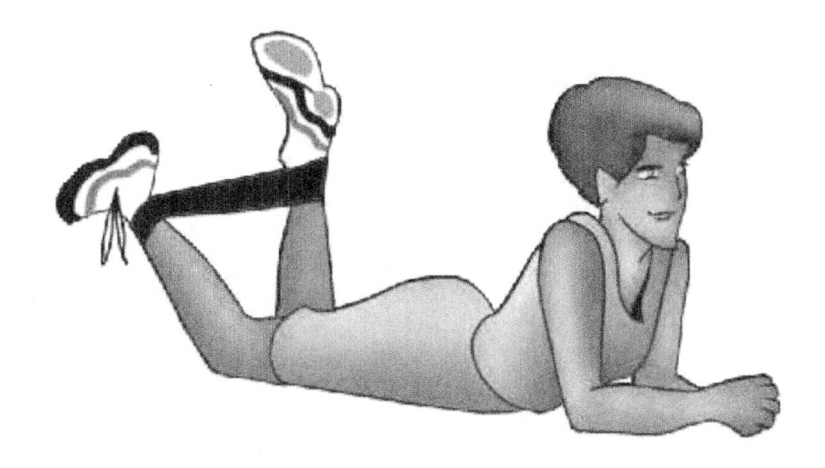

This sample, beginner-friendly resistance band workout program would be ideal for seniors. This workout program follows a circuit design, which means each exercise follows the other without any rests between them until you complete the entire set of exercises. Each circuit has ten exercises.

In the first week, you may perform just one circuit. In the second, you will have gained a little strength and will do one circuit, rest, and then do a second one. As you proceed through the weeks, add a circuit a week until you are strong enough to do four circuits a day.

NOTE: The numbers in bracket represent the number of times you should repeat the routine.

Beginner Workout Program

MON	TUES	WED	THURS	FRI
Band Push-Ups (10)	REST	Band Push-Ups (10)	REST	Band Push-Ups (10)
Band Squats (15)		Band Squats (15)		Band Squats (15)
Band Deadlift (15)		Band Deadlift (15)		Band Deadlift (15)
Mountain Climbers (15 each side)		Mountain Climbers (15 each side)		Mountain Climbers (15 each side)
Seated Shoulder Press (15)		Seated Shoulder Press (15)		Seated Shoulder Press (15)

Bicep Curl (15)		Bicep Curl (15)		Bicep Curl (15)
Triceps Extension (15)		Triceps Extension (15)		Triceps Extension (15)

Arthritis Workout Program

If you're battling arthritis, keep the following guidelines in mind when taking up exercise:

- If you feel more pain 2 hours after a workout than when you started, workout less next time.

- On some days, you won't feel like exercising. On such days, motivates yourself to work out for 5 minutes and recheck your mood.

- Do not exercise beyond what your body can take.

- Do not put unnecessary strain on a swollen joint. Leave it alone; do not exercise it.

- Do not use painkillers to cover up pain just because you want to keep exercising.

- Use light exercises to warm-up before any workout routine. You can also take a warm shower before a workout or ice any joints that may be problematic.

- To reduce pain, stick to movements within a joint's range motion, and maintain proper form throughout the exercise.

- As you progress, always consult your doctor to know which exercises you should do and which ones to avoid.

Below is a basic program you can use and improve on as you grow in your exercise journey.

Arthritis Workout Program

ARTHRITIS			
EXERCISE	**SETS**	**REP/TIME**	**REST**
Pull Down	1	6-12	30-45 seconds
Horizontal Chest Press	1	6-12	30-45 seconds
Frontal Raise	1	6-12	30-45 seconds
Triceps Extension	1	6-12	30-45 seconds

| Biceps Curl | 1 | 6-12 | 30-45 seconds |
| Gas Pedal | 1 | 6-12 | 30-45 seconds |

Back Pain Workout Program

If you suffer from lower back pain, keep the following guidelines in mind before taking up any exercise routine or program:

- If you feel more pain 2 hours after a workout than when you started, workout less next time.

- On some days, you won't feel like exercising. On such days, motivates yourself to work out for 5 minutes and recheck your mood.

- Do not exercise beyond what your body can take.

- Do not put unnecessary strain on a swollen joint. Leave it alone; do not exercise it.

- Do not use painkillers to cover up pain just because you want to keep exercising.

- Use light exercises to warm-up before any workout routine. You can also take a warm shower before a workout or ice any joints that may be problematic.

- To reduce pain, stick to movements within a joint's range motion, and maintain proper form throughout the exercise.

As you progress, always consult your doctor to know which exercises you should do and which ones to avoid.

Here's a basic program;

Back pain Workout Program

BACK PAIN			
EXERCISE	**SETS**	**REP/TIME**	**REST**
Pull Down	1	8-12	30-45 seconds
Horizontal Chest Press	1	8-12	30-45 seconds
Shoulder Press	1	8-12	30-45 seconds

| Triceps Extension | 1 | 8-12 | 30-45 seconds |
| Biceps Curl | 1 | 8-12 | 30-45 seconds |

Hip Issues Workout Program

If you're struggling with hip issues, keep the following guidelines in mind before taking up any exercise routine:

- Avoid bringing your knee too close to your chest.

- Avoid crossing your waistline when you move your leg in front or behind the other leg.

- When doing squats or leg presses, keep your hips, knees, and ankles in a straight line.

- Avoid full squats.

Below is a sample workout program:

Hip Issues Workout Program

HIPS ISSUES			
EXERCISE	**SETS**	**REP/TIME**	**REST**
Gas Pedal	1-2	8-12	30-45 seconds
Leg Press	1-2	8-12	30-45 seconds
Squat	1-2	8-12	30-45 seconds

Side Step	1-2	8-12	30-45 seconds
Side Bend	1-2	8-12	30-45 seconds

Knee Issues Workout Program

If you're working through knee issues, keep the following guidelines in mind before starting any workout program:

- Avoid having your knees and toes pointing in different directions.

- Avoid exercises that require you to rotate or twist your knees. Further, avoid twisting your body when you have your feet fixed on the ground.

- Never force your leg to over-straighten at the knee.

- Do not perform stretches that require you to bend your knees too much.

- Do not squat any lower than the level at which your thighs make a 90-degree angle.

- When stretching, keep your knees slightly bent.

- Do not let the knee bend forward past the toes.

- Never go past your range of motion.

__Knee issues Workout Program__

KNEE ISSUES			
EXERCISE	**SETS**	**REP/TIME**	**REST**
Squat	2-3	8-12	30-45 seconds
Forward Lunge	2-3	8-12	30-45 seconds

Leg Curl	2-3	8-12	30-45 seconds
Pelvic Lift	2-3	8-12	30-45 seconds

Osteoporosis Workout Program

When exercising with osteoporosis, keep the following guidelines in mind:

- Take extra care when bending forward or twisting.

- Be watchful and careful when lifting overhead.

- Maintain proper posture and body mechanics at all times.

Pair this basic starter program with a gentle walking program.

Osteoporosis Workout Program

OSTEOPOROSIS			
EXERCISE	**SETS**	**REP/TIME**	**REST**
Horizontal Chest Press	1-2	8-15	30-45 seconds
Triceps Extension	1-2	8-15	30-45 seconds

Leg Press	1-2	8-15	30-45 seconds
Forward Lunge	1-2	8-15	30-45 seconds

Shoulder Issues Workout Program

If you suffer from shoulder issues, keep the following guidelines in mind before taking up any exercise routine:

- Avoid exercises that require you to raise your hands above your head or any that causes pain.

- After exercising, apply ice to any place that hurts, but only if your doctor approves of it. However, remember that you should not feel more or extreme pain after exercising.

- Perform exercises that work the chest and shoulders.

- Take precautions when performing an exercise that requires you to raise your hand above your head.

- Loosen your shoulders, let them relax, and don't shrug.

- Pull your shoulder blades together when engaging in arm-based exercises.

- If you have tight shoulders, don't bend your back to compensate for your inflexibility.

- Perform stretches for your chest and shoulder area often

Shoulder Issues Workout Program

SHOULDER ISSUES			
EXERCISE	**SETS**	**REP/TIME**	**REST**
Long Row	1-2	5-7	30-45 seconds
Lateral Pull Down	1-2	5-7	30-45 seconds

Shrug	1-2	5-7	30-45 seconds
Reverse Flye	1-2	5-7	30-45 seconds

Diabetes Workout Program

If you have diabetes, keep the following tips in mind before taking up any exercise routine:

- Avoid exercises and activities that strain your feet.

- Perform warm-up and cool-down exercises for a bit longer. These periods are vital when transitioning from moderate exercise to rest, especially for people with diabetes

- Do not perform heavy and intense exercises.

- Train at a rate where you can still hold a conversation comfortably.

- Be mindful of your insulin levels.

- If you have had retinal issues in the past, seek advice from your doctor before you begin.

Diabetes Workout Program

DIABETES			
EXERCISE	**SETS**	**REP/TIME**	**REST**
Standing Frontal Raise	1-2	8-15	30-45 seconds
Gas Pedal	1-2	8-15	30-45 seconds

Biceps Curl	1-2	8-15	30-45 seconds
Triceps Extension	1-2	8-15	30-45 seconds

High Blood Pressure Program

If you suffer from high blood pressure, keep the following guidelines in mind before taking up any exercise routine:

- Prioritize muscular endurance over strength. The objective is to be able to do many reps with a lighter load as opposed to being able to do a few reps with a heavier load.

- If your blood pressure is above 160/90, consult your doctor before you begin resistance training.

- Take extra care when lifting your hands over your head during exercise.

- Always make sure you adequately warm-up and cool down. Issues like high or low blood pressure can have adverse effects if you start too hard and stop exercising abruptly.

- Take deep breaths as you exercise. Don't hold your breath.

- Consult your doctor about the effects your medication can have on exercise.

- Don't over-exercise. You are over-exercising if you cannot whistle during an exercise routine.

High Blood Pressure Workout Program

HIGH BLOOD PRESSURE			
EXERCISE	**SETS**	**REP/TIME**	**REST**
Seated Horizontal Chest Press	1-2	8-15	30-45 seconds
Seated Reverse Flye	1-2	8-15	30-45 seconds

Gas Pedal	1-2	8-15	30-45 seconds
Leg Press	1-2	8-15	30-45 seconds

Conclusion

If you eat well and exercise regularly, you can be healthy and fit enough to live a fulfilling, joyful life.

Printed in Great Britain
by Amazon